A NOTE TO FELLOW TE...

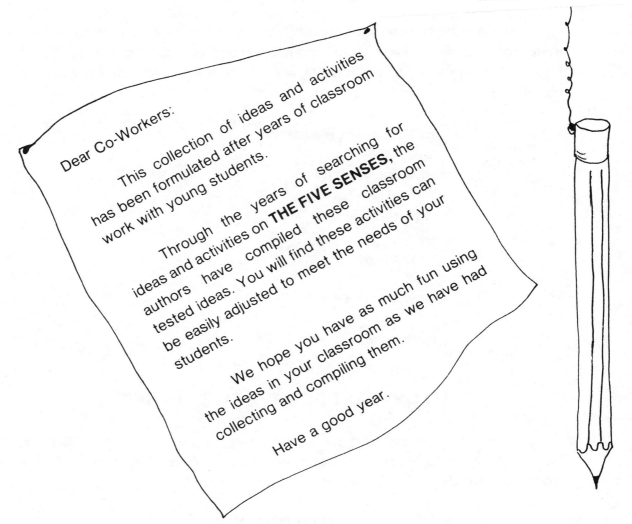

Dear Co-Workers:

This collection of ideas and activities has been formulated after years of classroom work with young students.

Through the years of searching for ideas and activities on **THE FIVE SENSES**, the authors have compiled these classroom tested ideas. You will find these activities can be easily adjusted to meet the needs of your students.

We hope you have as much fun using the ideas in your classroom as we have had collecting and compiling them.

Have a good year.

TABLE OF CONTENTS

Introduction....................... 1 - 6

Sense of Sight.................... 7 - 19

Sense of Hearing................20 - 33

Sense of Touch..................34 - 44

Sense of Taste...................45 - 53

Sense of Smell..................54 - 64

TESTING

PRETEST FOR THE FIVE SENSES

At the primary level, the pretesting situation will be very informal and depend largely on teacher evaluation. During large and small group discussions, answers to questions will indicate to the teacher whether or not the students are familiar with the concepts.

Examples of questions:

1. How do we see?

2. How do we hear?

3. How do we feel things?

4. How do we taste?

5. How do we smell things?

POST-TEST FOR THE FIVE SENSES

The post-testing will be more formal in that the students will be able to identify tastes, smells, textures, sounds, colors and shapes. Also, at the more difficult level, vocabulary words will be identified.

SCHEDULE

This unit is designed for the primary grades and designed to last about three weeks. The class schedule can be as follows:

Each of the five concepts in this unit will be three days in length.

1st day	The entire class
	Motivate interest through charts, filmstrips, stories and discussion.
2nd day	The entire class
	Experiments, field trips, experience stories.
3rd day	Small group activities.

KEEP A CHART

	KEEP A CHART	COLOR OF TOP I WORE	A NEW TASTE	A NEW TEXTURE I FELT	SOMETHING NICE I SAW	A SPECIAL SOUND	A NEW WORD I LEARNED
SUNDAY							
MONDAY							
TUESDAY							
WEDNESDAY							
THURSDAY							
FRIDAY							
SATURDAY							

CLASS RECORD FORM

completed tasks

NAME		1	2	3	4	5	6	7	8	9	10	11	12	13	14	15	16	17	18	19	20	21	22	23	24
	1																								
	2																								
	3																								
	4																								
	5																								
	6																								
	7																								
	8																								
	9																								
	10																								
	11																								
	12																								
	13																								
	14																								
	15																								
	16																								
	17																								
	18																								
	19																								
	20																								
	21																								
	22																								
	23																								
	24																								
	25																								
	26																								
	27																								
	28																								
	29																								
	30																								
	31																								
	32																								
	33																								
	34																								
	35																								
	36																								

POEM FOR THE FIVE SENSES

MY EYES CAN SEE

My eyes can see
My mouth can talk
My ears can hear
My feet can walk.

My nose can smell
My teeth can bite
My lids can flutter
My hand can write.

But when the sandman comes at night
Scatters sand
Turns out the light
I'll say "Good night"
To you and you
Each part of me says,
"Good night" too.

. . . Author Unknown

GROUP CONCEPTS TO BE DEVELOPED:

1. The senses inform us about the world around us.

2. We learn through using our senses - seeing, hearing, smelling, tasting and feeling.

3. Our senses help to tell us what goes on outside our body.

4. We use our senses to find things.

5. We use our senses to identify things.

6. We use our senses to solve problems.

ILLUSTRATE

Things I can feel.

Things I can see.

Things I can hear.

Things I can smell.

Things I can taste.

HOW DO WE SEE?

TOPIC CONCEPTS TO BE DEVELOPED:

1. We need light in order to see.

2. We see by using our eyes.

3. Seeing is one of our senses.

4. Our eyes enable us to see color and shape.

LARGE GROUP ACTIVITIES:

1. Have students identify the color as food coloring is added to small clear dishes of water. This can be done on the overhead projector.

2. Associate colors and feelings through a class discussion. What color makes one happy? What color makes one sad? What color makes a person cold? etc.

3. Allow each child to tell what his favorite color is and why.

4. Use a prism to show color. Demonstrate and discuss.

5. Listen to recordings about colors. A good album to use is **THE COLORS OF MY RAINBOW.** The album by Joe Wayman is available from Good Apple, Inc.

6. Read a story or poem about colors.

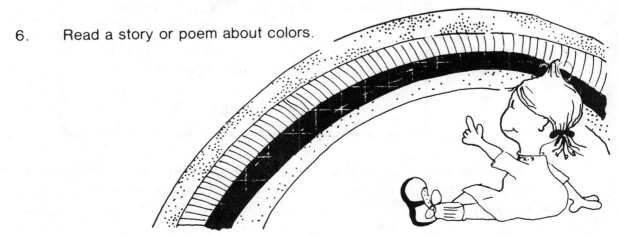

SMALL GROUP ACTIVITIES:

1. Have the children drop food coloring on folded white paper napkins. Observe the colors as they overlap.

2. Make dots with crayons on drawing paper. Overlap. Observe.

3. Make a tissue paper collage using paper of the three primary colors.

4. Cut colored construction paper into interesting shapes. Paste the shapes on large paper to create a design.

5. Play a matching game to identify the eight basic colors and the basic shapes.

6. Use coat hangers and basic shapes of various colors to create a mobile. Allow each student to contribute his favorite shape in his favorite color. Shapes can be made of construction paper or poster board.

7. Spend a day wearing cellophane glasses. Each child gets to wear glasses of each color for one hour.

COLORS

Blue is the color we see in the sky.
Black is the color of the tiny fly.

Brown is the color of the mountain bear.
Yellow is the color of a juicy pear.

Orange is the color of oranges we eat.
Green is the color of the grass on my street.

Purple is the color we see on the grapes.
Red is the color of the bullfighter's cape.

. . . Author Unknown

This poem may be duplicated for the children. After reading and discussing the poem, the children may want to write additional lines or illustrate each verse and make a book.

MULTICOLORED GLASSES

Duplicate this pattern so that each student can have a pair of glasses. Paste colored cellophane on the glasses for lenses. After cutting out the duplicated copy each child could color the frames of his glasses. To make the glasses more durable, laminate when completed.

MAKE A MOBILE

Connect the matching color words.

Name _____

red	ORANGE
brown	RED
green	BLACK
yellow	GREEN
blue	PURPLE
white	BROWN
orange	YELLOW
black	BLUE
purple	WHITE

Use the color shapes to make a mobile. One large mobile can be made by the class. Each child could contribute his favorite colored shape. Use a coat hanger and fishing line to create the mobile.

COLOR AND SHAPE

DOMINO GAME

Color each shape on the domino sheets. Inside each shape you will find letters indicating what color to color the shape. Then carefully cut out each domino. Select a classmate and play "The Color and Shape Domino Game."

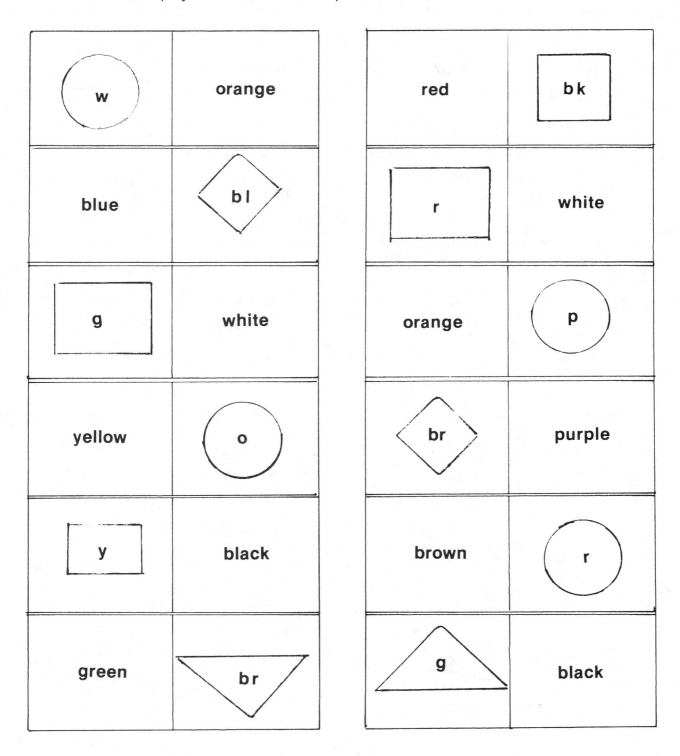

COLOR AND SHAPE DOMINO GAME cont.

COLOR AND SHAPE DOMINO GAME cont.

purple	r (rectangle)
bl (square)	blue
brown	bk (triangle)
w (circle)	red
orange	o (rectangle)
p (triangle)	yellow
white	g (circle)

br (triangle)	orange
red	y (triangle)
bl (circle)	white
green	bk (square)
y (rectangle)	blue
brown	r (circle)
o (square)	green

12

(o)	white	purple	[y]
purple	△ g	(p)	red
[b l]	black	yellow	[bk]
brown	▽ w	△ o	blue
(w)	yellow	orange	[br]
green	[r]	(p)	green
◇ y	red	black	▽ w

COLOR WHEEL

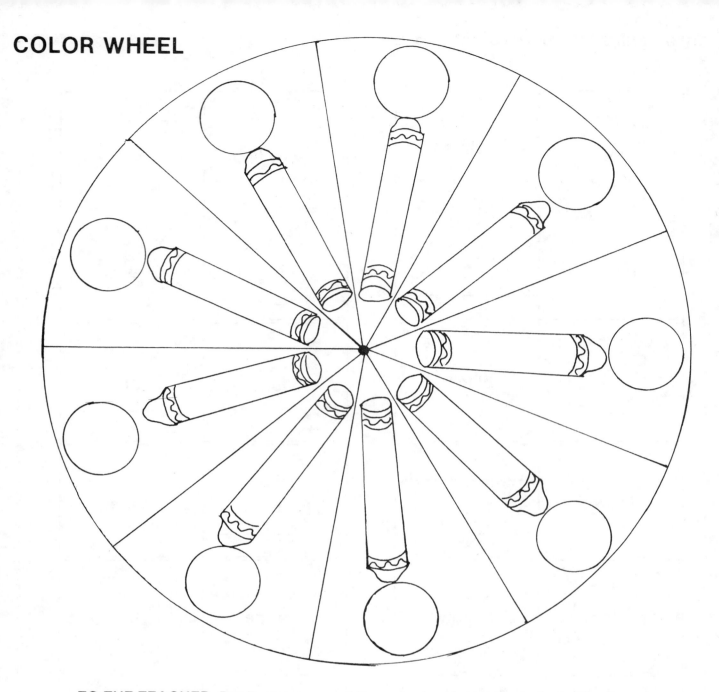

TO THE TEACHER: Duplicate a copy of the color key for each student. Direct each student to color each dot a color of his choice. Red, white, orange, yellow, blue, green, purple, black and brown are the colors that should be used. Then have each child print the appropriate color word in each triangle. Finally the child should cut out the color wheel.

Provide matching colored clothespins. You can make them easily by spray painting several pins each color. The color wheel could also be mounted on a piece of sturdy cardboard. Each child then clips the clothespin to the appropriate area of the color wheel.

This can be made self-checking by placing the same number on the back of the clothespin and the back of each section of the color wheel.

Color each shape on the left side of the paper according to the color word. Then color the umbrella by matching the colored triangles to the spaces on the umbrella. Cut out each shape and paste it in the correct position on the umbrella.

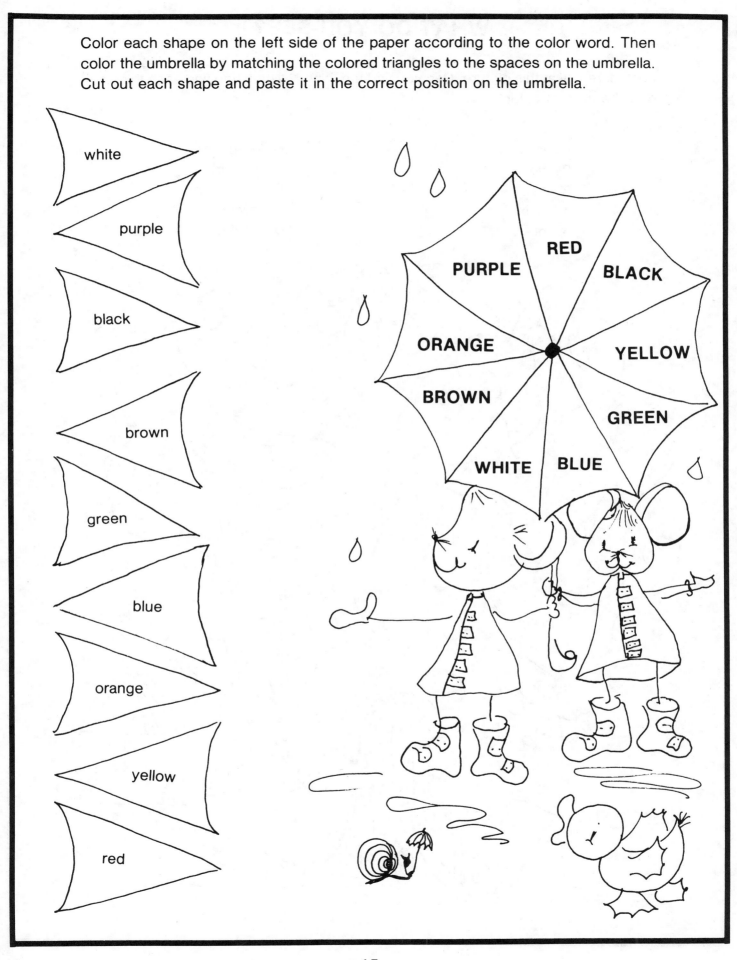

WHAT DO YOU SEE?

Look carefully at this picture. Can you find ten things? When you find each thing color it the correct color.

1. lamp
2. hen
3. fish
4. iron
5. glove

6. elephant
7. flower
8. hat
9. hammer
10. pitcher

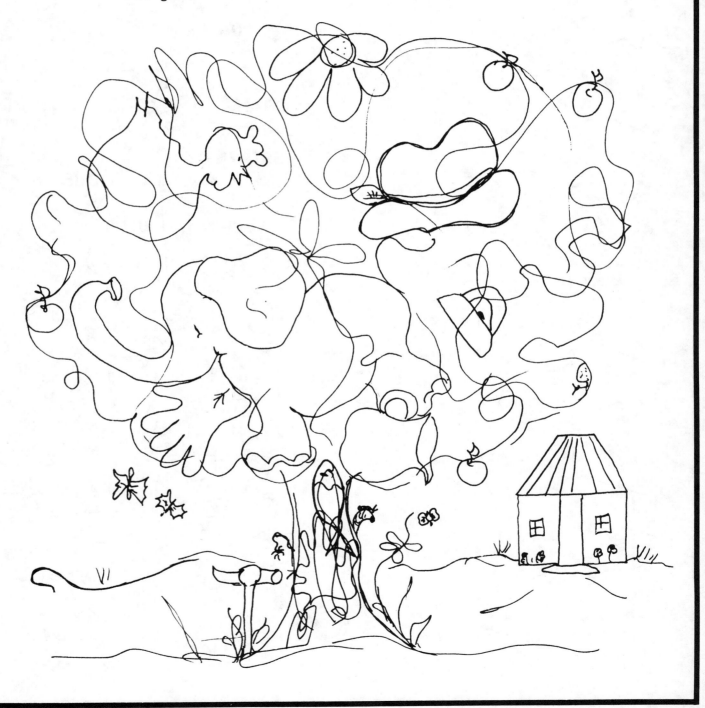

16

How many things
can you make with a circle?

How many things
can you make with a diamond?

How many things
can you make with a square?

How many things can you
make with a rectangle?

17

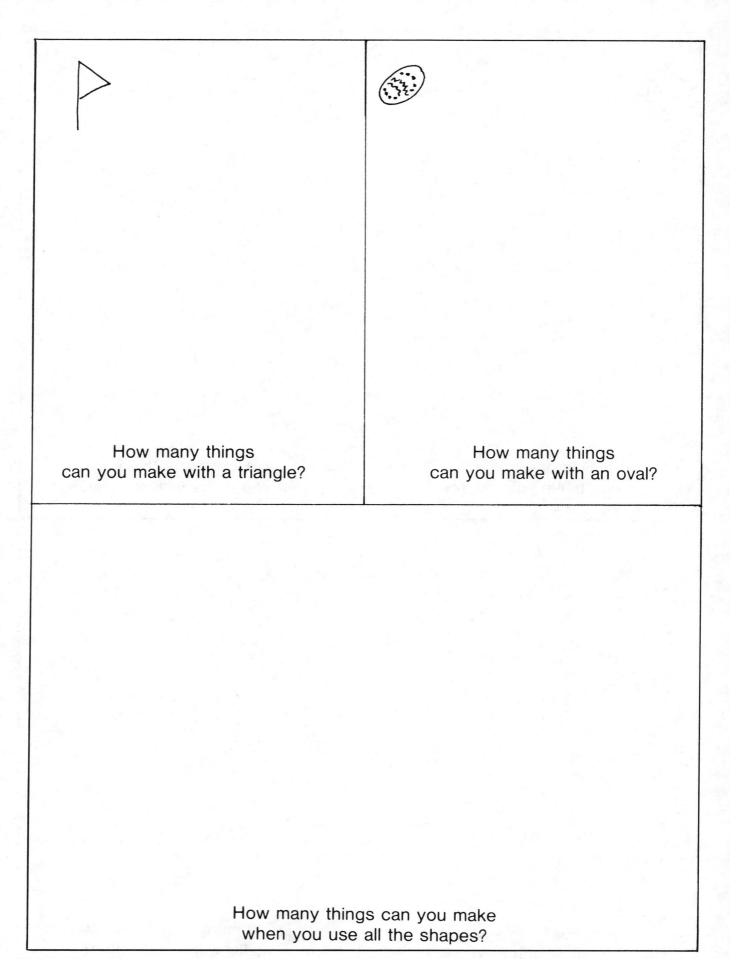

How many things
can you make with a triangle?

How many things
can you make with an oval?

How many things can you make
when you use all the shapes?

FIND OUT BY LOOKING

Place several objects on a table. The objects are to be sorted according to color, and then the learner should place the correct color word card with each group.

Objects that could be used include:

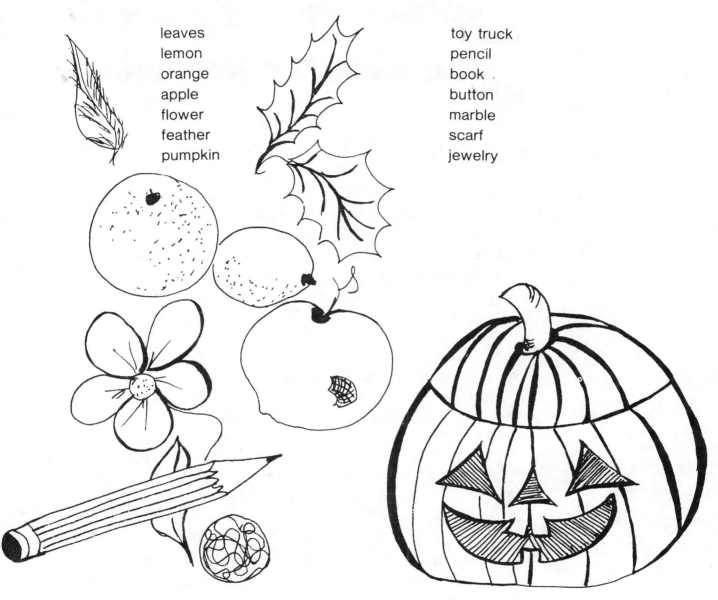

leaves	toy truck
lemon	pencil
orange	book .
apple	button
flower	marble
feather	scarf
pumpkin	jewelry

The color cards can be made by printing the color word with appropriate color of crayon on a 3" x 5" index card.

After students have mastered sorting the objects that are basic colors (green, blue, yellow, orange, red, black, purple, brown and white) introduce other colors such as pink, tan, silver, etc.

HOW DO WE HEAR?

TOPIC CONCEPTS TO BE DEVELOPED:

1. The ears are the sense organ that makes it possible for hearing to take place.

2. It is possible to observe carefully with the ears as well as the eyes.

3. It is possible to recognize the source of sound when it cannot be seen.

LARGE GROUP ACTIVITIES:

1. Play "The Talking Objects" game. If a garage could talk, what story would it tell? What sounds would it make?

2. Follow directions given by the teacher. The teacher gives a direction and the students follow. An example would be, "Raise your left hand." The directions can increase in length to increase listening skills.

3. Listen to a tape recording of sounds. The students should try to identify each sound as it is heard.

4. Play "The Secret Game." Directions follow in this section of activities.

5. Read some books and poems about sounds. You will be able to find a story where the students can make sounds as the words are heard.

6. Invite a musician into the classroom to demonstrate the sounds of several musical instruments. Students can then play rhythm instruments, make musical instruments and create body movements to various sounds and rhythms.

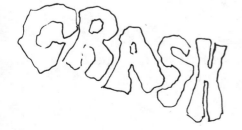
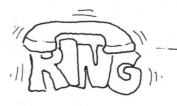
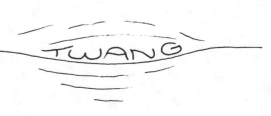

7.   For a field trip visit the high school band while it is practicing. Take a trip to a telephone company or to a class for the hearing impaired.

8.   Pop corn. Listen to all the sounds. Eat and enjoy. Don't forget the sounds of eating.

9.   Have a doctor visit the classroom. Explain about a stethoscope. Listen to heartbeats.

SMALL GROUP ACTIVITIES:

1.   On a table place a variety of materials that can be used to make sounds. An eggbeater, cotton balls, alarm clock, seashell, comb, aluminum foil, plastic silverware, pans, whistle, etc., can be included. Each child after experimenting can create the sound he likes best. The class can try to identify what is making the sound.

2.   Walk in the hallway with a tape recorder and record five interesting sounds. Bring the tape back to the classroom and have the students identify the sounds. The students will enjoy using the tape recorder. The tape recorder could be sent home with the students or given to them during a recess or lunch period. Who can record the most unusual sound?

3.   Set up a listening center in your classroom. Provide a variety of tapes and records. Many of the recordings should be stories. Using headphones each child should listen to one story or song and then in turn relate what was heard to the class.

4.   Make a class "sound" mobile. Use pieces of wood, bells, buttons, tin cans, sheets of aluminum foil, etc.

HEARING - EARS

The bells ring loud,
Both far and near,
Draw a picture of
What your ears hear.

SOUND PICTURES

Make a picture to describe each sound word.

creaking	scratch
plop	gurgle
splat	squeak
howl	plunk

SOUNDS I LIKE TO HEAR

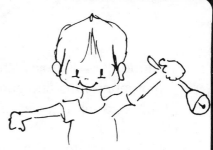

SOUNDS I DO NOT LIKE TO HEAR

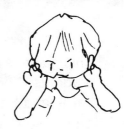

LISTENING GAME

Students will enjoy this easy-to-make listening game. You will need some empty margarine tubs and some word and picture cards. These cards can be made by cutting index cards to a size that will easily fit on top of the tubs.

Inside each tub place an object that will make some sound (great or small) when the tub is shaken. When the sound is identified its matching picture and word card should be placed on the lid of the tub.

Possible ideas to be placed in the tubs might include:

buttons   wad of paper
gravel   paper clip
sand   candy
cotton balls   ½ cup of flour
eraser   bottle cap
coins   nail
ball

THE TALKING OBJECTS GAME

This game is a good language development game as well as a listening game for young students. The unfinished sentences, similar to those below, can be printed on index cards and be drawn from a brightly decorated box. This game can be used as a large group, small group or individual activity.

1.   If a garage could talk what story would it tell?

2.   If a rug could talk what would it say to your feet?

3.   If flowers could talk what would they say to the sun?

4.   If your garbage could talk what would it say?

5.   If your pencil could tell a story what story would it tell?

The children's stories/answers could be recorded on a tape to be played back at a later time to encourage expansion of the basic answer. Or, the answers could be recorded on paper by a parent or student helper and each student could then illustrate his response. Completed work could be hung about the classroom for all to enjoy.

PAPER CUP TELEPHONE

MATERIALS:
2 paper
cups
1 piece of
string
2 buttons
a nail

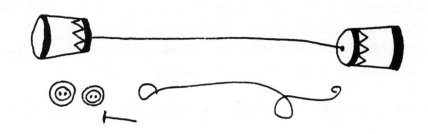

DIRECTIONS:

1. Use the nail to punch holes in the bottoms of the two paper cups.

2. Push the ends of the strings through the holes in the paper cups.

3. Thread string through the holes. Tie the buttons to the ends of the string.

4. Pull strings tight and speak into the cup.

RIDDLES - WHAT MAKES THIS SOUND?

These riddles and others that you find should be read, listened to, illustrated and enjoyed. After reading several riddles to the students ask them to share one they know with their classmates. The children's riddles can be recorded for further listening and enjoyment.

Crackle, crackle.
I help keep you warm
        in winter or on a camp-out.
Crackle, crackle, crackle.
What makes this sound?

Bang, bang, bang.
This sound happens when Daddy
        builds a house for my puppy.
Bang, bang, bang.
What makes this sound?

Hum-m-m, hum-m-m.
I help mother clean the house.
Hum-m-m, hum-m-m.
What makes this sound?

Mew, mew, mew.
I am soft and fuzzy.
Purr, purr, purr.
What makes this sound?

THE SECRET GAME

Whisper a secret to a student, such as Susie likes to jump. The student, in turn, whispers the secret to the next student. This continues until all students participating in the activity have listened to the secret and passed it on to another player. The originator of the secret should be the last to hear the secret. This person reveals the secret to all and compares the final statement with the beginning sentence.

Each secret-passing attempt should be followed by a discussion of what happened.

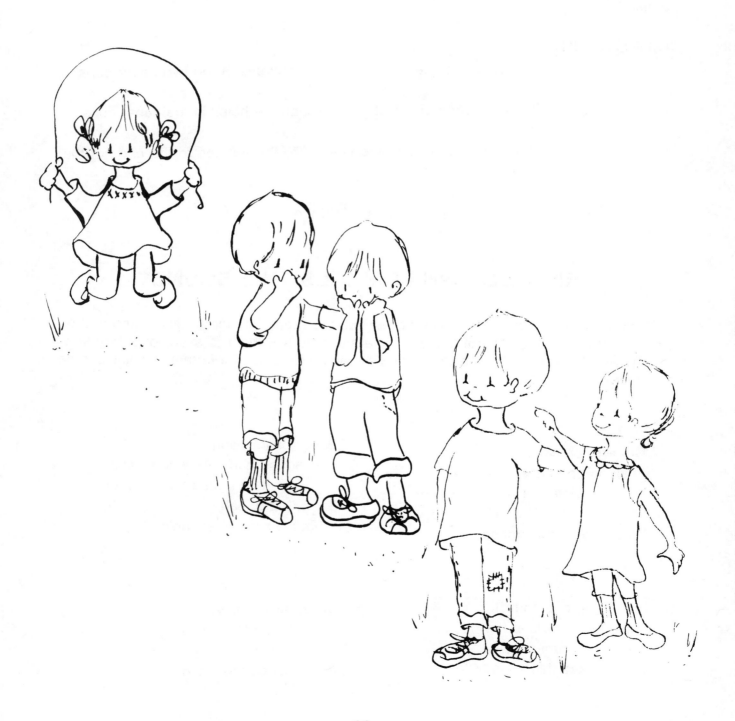

WHO AM I?   WHAT AM I?

This activity is recommended as a small group activity. Picture or word cards can be made from index cards and drawn from a small box.

To play, the child without showing the card to anyone, imitates the object. The next turn is decided by the child giving the correct answer to the imitation.

Provide some blank cards. After a small group of students have played the game, allow each player to design an additional card to be included in the game.

Some cards are provided for you on this page and the next two.

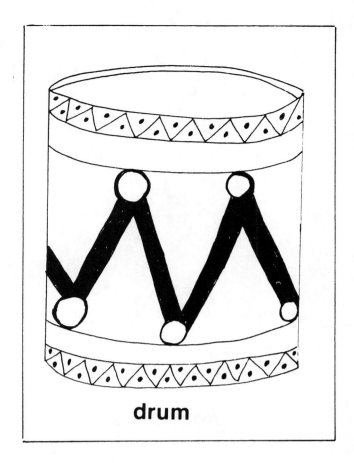

drum

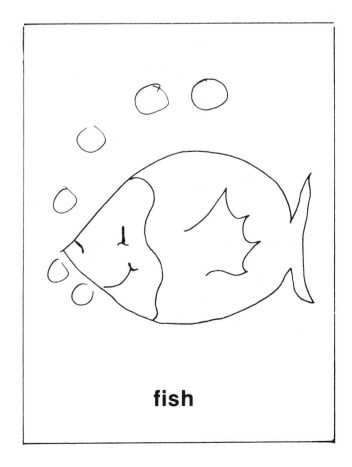

fish

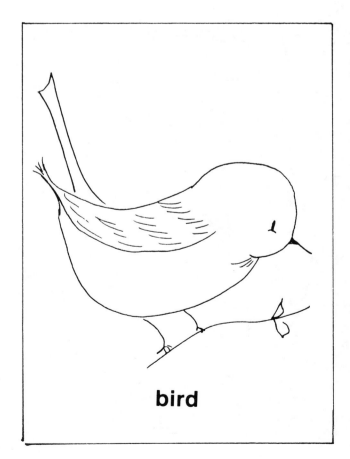

bird

27

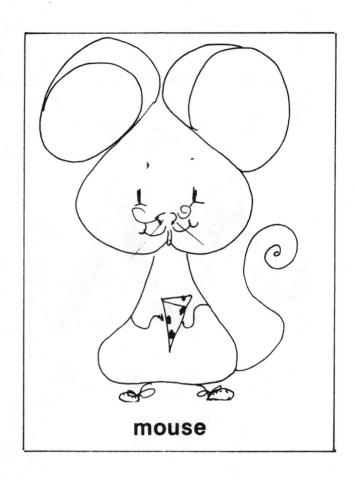

mouse

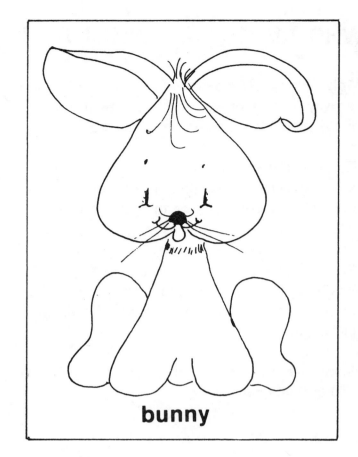

bunny

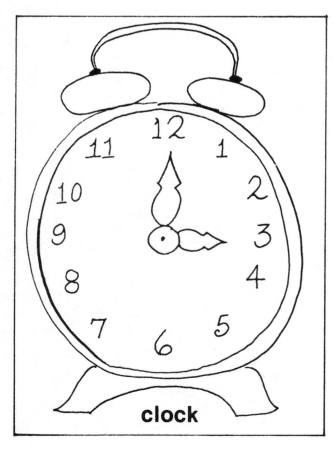

clock

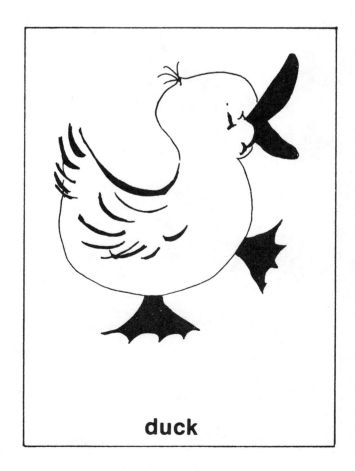

duck

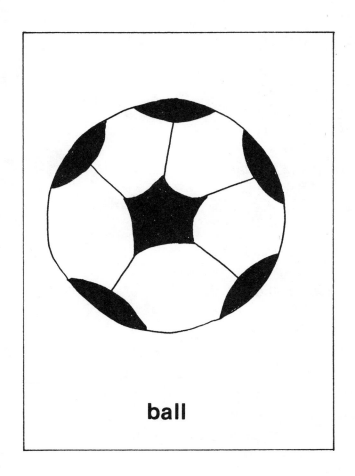

ball

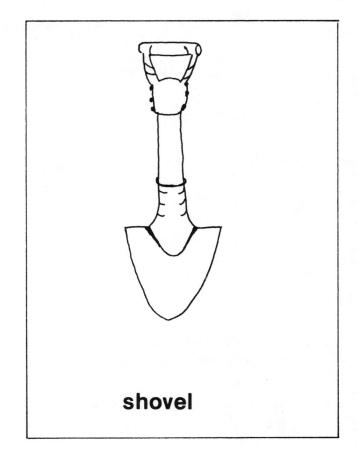

shovel

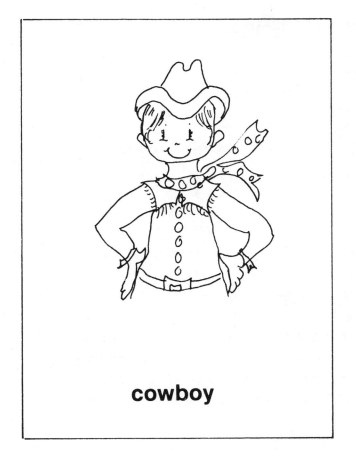

cowboy

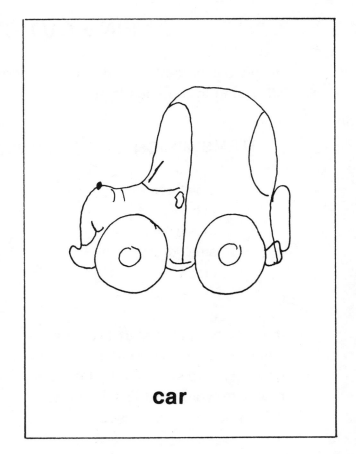

car

CHART OF SOUNDS

sounds of summer	sounds of spring
sounds of winter	sounds of fall
sounds of school	sounds of the farm
sounds of home	sounds of the city
sounds of animals	sounds of machines
sounds of people	sounds of the night

From sheets of paper create a large chart. Each section or each sheet of paper should be titled with one of the above headings. After an introductory classroom discussion, the children may cut pictures from old magazines and paste them in the appropriate areas of the chart. Children could draw additional pictures in the proper areas of the chart. The teacher could then label each picture with the word.

FIND OUT BY LISTENING

Blindfold a student. The student will identify sounds by listening. Take the blindfold off. Listen to the sounds again and match to the correct word cards.

ITEMS WHICH MAKE SOUNDS	WORD CARDS
small bell	bell
playground whistle	whistle
music triangle	triangle
small drum	drum
clock	clock

It would be fun to start this game by having the blindfolded student listen to the voices of some classmates. Five classmates saying five different words might be a good place to start. When the blindfold has been removed the player gives the appropriate word card to the student who said the word. The number of people involved could be increased.

LOUD OR QUIET?

Fill in the blank with the correct word, **loud** or **quiet**.

1.   A car horn is _____.

2.   Falling leaves make a _____ sound.

3.   A paintbrush makes a _____ sound.

4.   The rock band has a _____ sound.

5.   Fireworks make a _____ sound.

6.   The kitten is very _____.

7.   A ticking clock is _____.

8.   The alarm on a clock is _____.

9.   I like the television when it is _____.

10.   The _____ made a _____ sound.

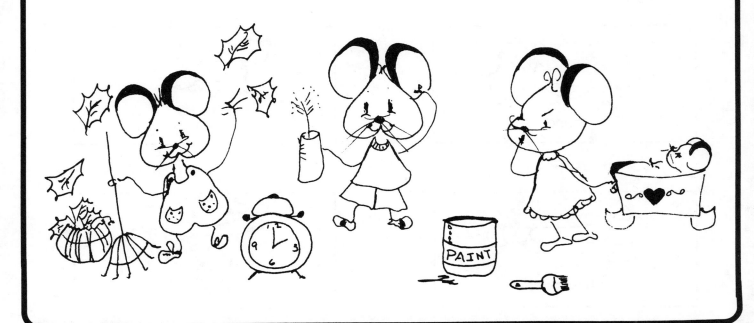

SOUNDS TO CUT AND PASTE

Cut and paste these pictures into the correct column on the following page.

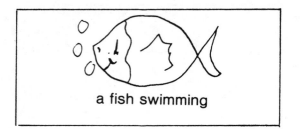

a fish swimming

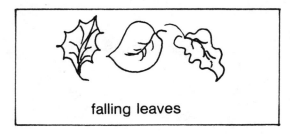

falling leaves

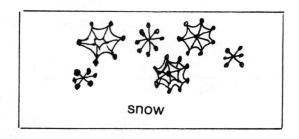

snow

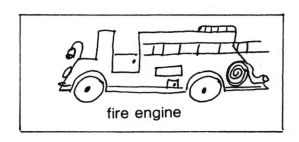

fire engine

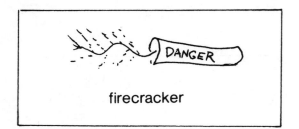

firecracker

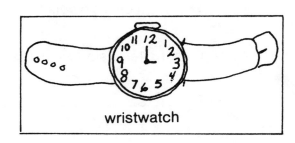

wristwatch

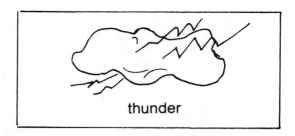

thunder

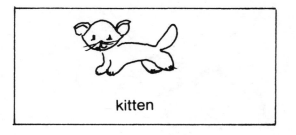

kitten

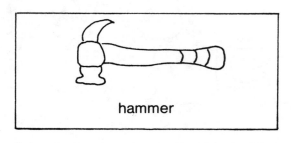

hammer

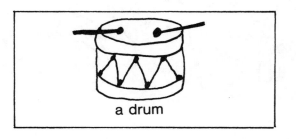

a drum

LOUD SOUNDS   **QUIET SOUNDS**

HOW DO WE FEEL THINGS?

TOPIC CONCEPTS TO BE DEVELOPED:

1. The sense of feeling, or touch is a source of information.

2. The sense of feeling tells us whether objects are hard or soft, rough or smooth, sharp or dull, hot or cold.

3. The sense of feeling gives us information about shape and about size.

4. The skin is the organ of the sense of feeling.

LARGE GROUP ACTIVITIES:

1. Walk outside. Touch many things that you see. Touch as many textures as you can. With paper and chalk make texture rubbings.

2. Create a rebus story. The teacher can begin the story and the students can contribute ideas.

3. Read a variety of books and poems about feeling/touching to the class. A short film or filmstrip could also be shown.

4. Have a touch hunt. Take an "in-school" field trip. Walk about the school touching and discussing the textures of various items. Why do they have so many textures?

5. Invite a blind person to the classroom. Discuss how books in Braille are printed and used. The local librarian may be able to help. The blind visitor can tell about the development of his sense of touch.

SMALL GROUP ACTIVITIES:

1. Make "feely" bags. Students identify objects in the bags using only the sense of touch. Discussions can follow.

2. Have each student make a collection of things he likes to touch. The child can put the items in a paper bag and place his name on the outside. These can be placed about the room and other children can reach inside and find out what classmates have included.

3. Make "touchy" letters. Kinnesthic alphabet cards can help many students to learn and be able to print the alphabet. Use stencils to trace the shapes of the various letters on pieces of light cardboard. The students can glue sand on the outlined areas. When dry, the children can touch the letter shape while saying its name. The children will enjoy trying to name each letter using only their sense of touch for identification.

4. Use modeling clay to create letters and numbers. It can also be used to create miniatures of common objects. Students could then try to identify these objects by touch.

5. A classroom sandbox is a great place for students to play, work and learn.

6. Make a touch mobile. After completion, blindfold a child and have him identify the various textures.

clothes hanger	aluminum foil
string and yarn	straws
cotton balls	paper clips
sandpaper	buttons
scraps of material	ricrac
spoons (plastic/wooden)	twigs/bark
paper cups	dried weeds
corrugated cardboard	hair/fur

7. Describe how an animals's coat feels. Students'responses may vary. One child may choose to describe a snake's skin while another may describe a kitten's fur.

8. Collect a variety of materials. Make a texture collage. Each child may contribute something.

9. Do some finger painting.

10. Play "Blind Man's Bluff" or "Pin the Tail on the Donkey." Better yet develop an educational version of either game and play it.

11. Paint with whipped soap. Have the students draw a picture on a large sheet of construction paper. Then paint it with the soap mixture.

    Mix a granular soap with water (a few drops at a time). Use an electric mixer, set on whip, to blend. Mix till the soap becomes fluffy like marshmallow. Food color or tempera paint may be added if color is desired.

12. For a craft project make a cereal or a pasta mosaic.

HOT OR COLD? AN EXPERIMENT

You will need three bowls of water, one hot (but, not too hot), one warm and one cold.

Put one hand in the hot water and one hand in the cold water. Then, quickly put both hands in the warm water. What happens? Allow each child to try this.

The cold hand feels hot and the hot hand feels cold.

Place an ice cube in each bowl. Students can time how long it takes each cube to melt. To add more excitement to this experiment have the ice cubes colored a bright red (food coloring). Students will enjoy watching the surrounding water change colors as the ice cubes melt.

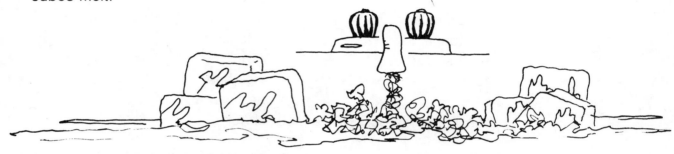

LEAF RUBBINGS

Select several different shaped leaves. Place a leaf under paper and color gently on top of it. You will see the veins of the leaf and its shape appear.

Mount the completed drawings on pieces of brightly colored construction paper and hang about the classroom. The owner's name could be printed below the picture and the picture could be taped to the front of the owner's desk.

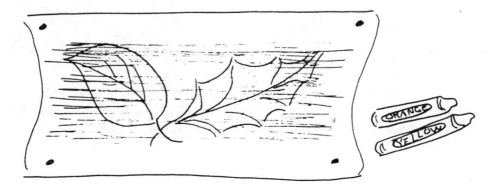

TOUCH AND LOOK

Label six boxes with one of the following words:

smooth	round	rough
flat	hard	soft

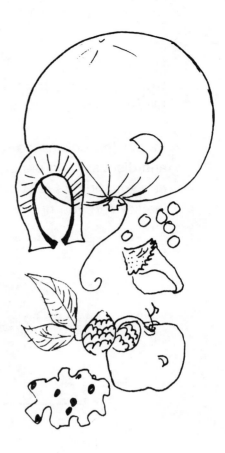

Sort the following items into the labeled boxes.

pine cone	rock	marble
piece of fur	magnet	inflated balloon
sponge	apple	seashell
soft clay	feather	piece of paper

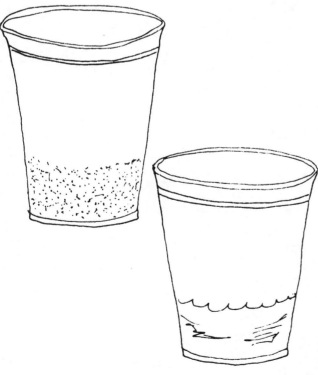

WET OR DRY

AN EXPERIMENT

Pour an inch of sand into one paper cup and an inch of water into another. Let the child without looking, put his finger into each cup. Then, discuss. Ask questions.

1. Is the material rough or smooth?

2. Is the material cool or warm?

3. Is the material in small or large pieces?

4. Is it a liquid?

Many children will be able to identify both materials.

FEELING COLLAGE

Cut out pictures from old magazines and make a collage. When paste is dry use a black crayon or felt marker to trace around a child's hand.

Mount the collage hand prints on contrasting construction paper. Use for display and discussion groups. What kind of things can you touch with your fingers? What can your fingers tell you? Are there some things that you can not touch? What information can you not get by just touching an item (color, taste, etc.)?

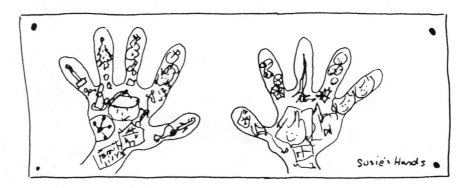

BLIND MAN GAME

Find out by touching.

Place several objects on a table. Blindfold a student. Place objects one at a time in the student's hand and ask for identification.

Suggested items for identification:

piece of fur	piece of sponge
inflated balloon	bar of soap
pine cone	bottle cap
lump of sugar	pill bottle
a 45 rpm record	book of matches
an orange	stick of celery
peanut in shell	

HOW TO MAKE "FEELLY" BAGS

Pin this pattern to two thicknesses of material. Stitch around the curved edge with the right sides together. Next turn down the open end and hem. Run a cord in the opening to make a drawstring tie.

Hide small objects inside the **"FEELLY" BAGS** for the children to touch and identify. Your students will have fun with this game.

The material used to make these "feelly" bags could be a bright colored and bold patterned material. If several bags are made glue a swatch of each material to a piece of poster board. Word cards or picture cards can be made and the students can place each card under the appropriate swatch of fabric.

IDEAS FOR "FEELLY" OBJECTS

piece of cotton   key

wood block   plastic glass

shoestring   small stuffed toy

Ping-Pong ball   tree bark

marble

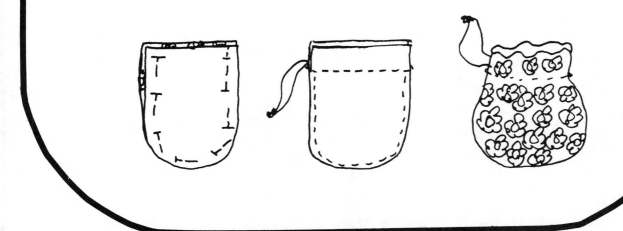

TOUCHING - HANDS

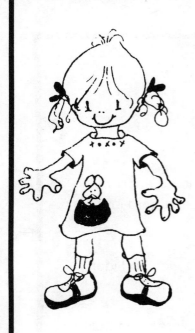

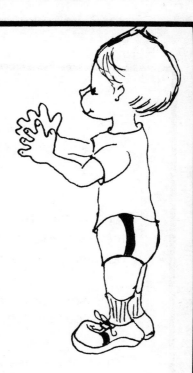

My hands can clap,

My fingers can wiggle,

Touching furry animals,

Can make me giggle.

Draw an animal you would like to touch.

MATCH THE OPPOSITES

Stretch your vocabulary with these touch words. Can you match the opposites?
Draw a line to connect each pair of opposites.

hard	hurt
wet	soft
tickle	dry
bumpy	smooth

smooth	stiff
flexible	rough
silky	cold
hot	scratchy

sticky	cool
flat	slippery
fuzzy	fluffy
warm	slick

sharp	dull
slick	silky
wooly	clean
coarse	rough

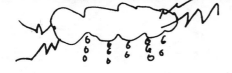

41

CEREAL MOSAIC

You will need a round or puffed type of cereal, small pie tins, glue, construction paper and pencil.

On the construction paper, lightly draw a simple picture. Each child is to add glue to the picture where pieces are to be placed.

The picture can be more colorful if colored pieces of cereal are used.

While waiting for the glue to dry, the clean-up activities can take place.

When children are showing their creations to other classmates, some cereal may be served as a snack and as a reward for a good clean job.

This activity can be done with a variety of pastas.

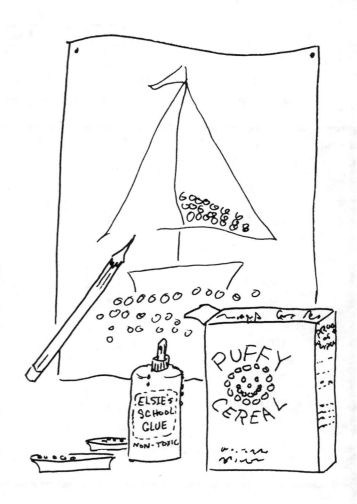

STRAW CRAFT

You will need seven to ten straws per child, construction paper, glue, scissors and crayons.

Younger children will enjoy just arranging the straws in a design. Older students may want to first draw a picture on the construction paper and then fill in the spaces with pieces of straw. Use crayons to color in the background of the picture.

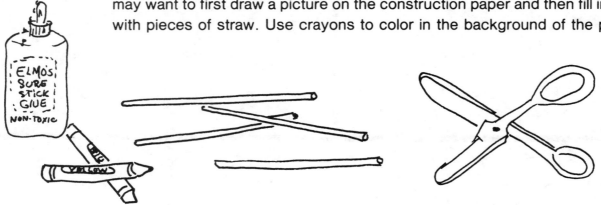

LET'S PRETEND

As well as being a tool for developing awareness of listening this activity is a good tool for language development. The students pull question cards out of a box. Questions should be answered with the idea that the object is actually in the classroom and the students could touch the object mentioned in the question. To play, a student draws a card from the box and asks classmates to answer. The more answers the better. Of course, there are no correct answers.

1. How would a star feel?

2. How would a monster feel?

3. How would an alligator feel?

4. How would a dinosaur feel?

5. How would a cloud feel?

6. How would a giant's nose feel?

7. How would the top of a mountain feel?

8. How would the bottom of the ocean feel?

9. How would moon dust feel?

10. How would a zebra's tail feel?

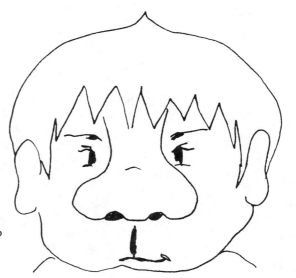

VOCABULARY WHEEL

The vocabulary wheel can be made from a pizza wheel or the pattern on the following page can be cut out and glued to a piece of cardboard.

Divide the wheel into sections and place a texture, to be identified in each section. On wooden, clip clothespins print the descriptive words.

Students should clip the clothespins to the corresponding section of the wheel. Words for the clothespins could include:

cold	itchy	hot	hard
soft	slick	wet	smooth

VOCABULARY WHEEL PATTERN

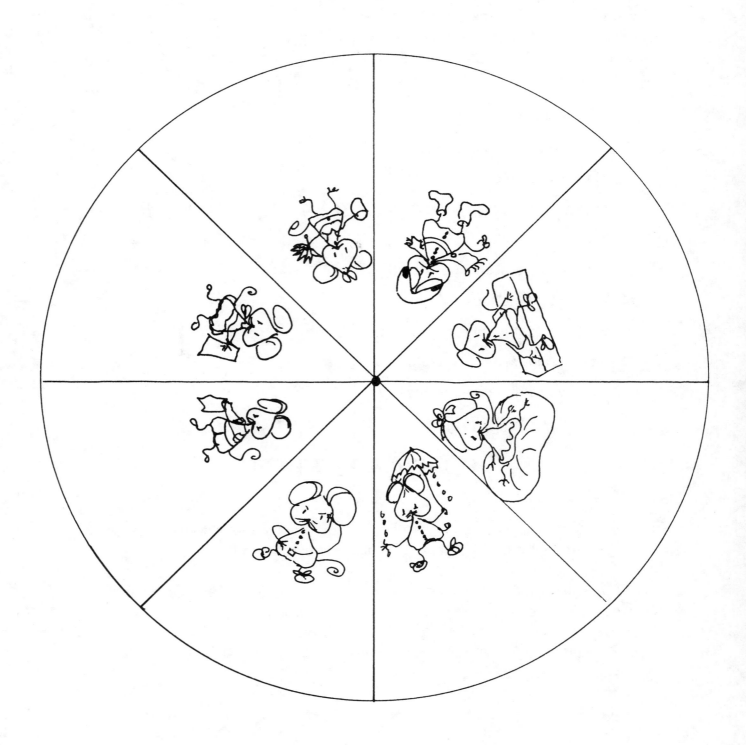

HOW DO WE TASTE THINGS?

TOPIC CONCEPTS TO BE DEVELOPED:

1. The tongue is the organ of taste.

2. The sense of smell is closely connected with the sense of taste.

3. It is much easier to identify flavors if one can smell a food as well as taste it.

LARGE GROUP ACTIVITIES:

1. Take a field trip to a local supermarket and bakery. Observe various kinds of foods (meats, vegetables, fruits, baked goods). Observe some unfamiliar foods. Can you imagine the taste?

2. Have a tasting party. Invite another class to join your children. Each child should be encouraged to taste a little bit of everything. Include salty, sweet, bitter and sour items in those you taste.

3. During storytime read books and poems about taste.

4. Play the "Lifesaver" game. Close eyes, put Lifesaver in mouth. Can the flavor be guessed? Make a graph showing how many students could identify each flavor. Why were some flavors easier to identify?

5. Invite someone from the community who was born and raised in a foreign country to your classroom. This person will most likely be able to bring some new tastes to your classroom for your students to try.

SMALL GROUP ACTIVITIES:

1. Use the sense of sight and the sense of taste and categorize picture cards of food according to color and taste.

2. Use old magazines to find pictures of foods you would like to taste. Each child could make a collage of pictures. All efforts could be bound together in a book.

3. Make a mouth collage. Attach a large sheet of paper to a wall space. Each student can search for pictures of mouths, cut them out and glue them to the paper. Student drawings could also be accepted.

4. Create a variety of matching games involving the sense of taste.

5. Explain that the tongue can only taste four things, sweet, sour, bitter and salt. Then ask students a variety of questions. If the tongue can only taste four things how can we tell the difference between strawberry ice cream and vanilla ice cream? (By the smell of the ice cream as well as by the appearance.)

6. Play the three games described in this section: What's On the Tray?, Fill the Pockets, Size and Shape.

7. Make peanut butter. Place roasted peanuts in a meat grinder or blender. Mix with a little butter. Spread on crackers and enjoy.

8. Paint with pudding and of course eat the leftovers.

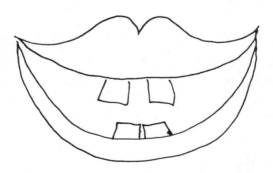

SAUCE! SAUCE! APPLESAUCE!

Ask each child to bring one apple to school for a very special day, Applesauce Day.

Under the close supervision of the teacher, let each child cut the apple into four pieces. (Include some discussion of the words whole, half, and fourth.)

Depending upon the age of the child, let him peel his apple and core it. If desired the apples could be washed and cooked- peeling, seeds, core, and all.

Cook the apples over medium heat, stirring (each child should have a turn) from time to time until they are squishy. Do not add water unless the mixture seems too dry. Fresh apples will usually have enough juice of their own.

If the apples were peeled and cored, add a little honey if you would like them to be sweeter. A little lemon juice will bring out the tart flavor. Sprinkle on a bit of cinnamon, if desired, and enjoy.

If the apples were cooked with the peelings on, they will need to be put through a food mill before adding the honey, lemon and cinnamon.

During this entire process point out changes that take place and how the various senses are constantly playing an important role in the learning process. Discuss the texture of the unpeeled, the peeled, the cooked apple. Discuss the smell of the apple while it is being peeled and cooked. Discuss the sounds that occur while the apple is being peeled, cored, and cooked.

TASTE SOME PUMPKIN SEEDS

When carving a Halloween pumpkin, be sure and save the seeds for a delicious treat.

First, wash the seeds to get rid of any pumpkin strings that might be stuck to them. Put the seeds on a paper towel and pat them dry. Spread them on a cookie sheet.

Pour melted butter or vegetable oil over the seeds. Sprinkle on some salt. You may want to put the seeds into a bowl before you add the butter and salt so the mixing will be easier and the coating even.

Put the seeds in an oven set at 300 degrees for about half an hour or until they are golden brown and crispy.

SORTING GAME - SIZE AND SHAPE

Place several kinds of vegetables and fruits on a table. The children will sort the foods and place them on the correct mat. Each mat should have a statement stapled to it. The mats can be made from pieces of cardboard.

Statements could include:

Kinds of foods to include on the table:

1. It is little.
2. It is round.
3. It is oval.
4. It is long.
5. It is leafy.
6. It is hard.
7. It is sweet.
8. It is bitter.
9. It is orange.
10. It is green and soft.
11. It is red and hard.

carrot	tangerine	squash
onion	strawberry	grapefruit
orange	celery	cabbage
lemon	lettuce	green bean
cucumber	apple	beet
banana	pear	tomato
peach	plum	potato
avocado	grapes	spinach
mushroom	strawberry	lime

FILL THE POCKETS

On a sheet of poster board place title, "Fill the Pockets" and four pockets labeled as shown below. The pockets can be made of construction paper and glued to the sheet of poster board.

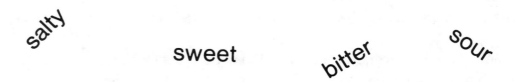

On index cards that will easily slip into the pockets, glue pictures of foods or print the names of foods. The student sorts the cards placing each card in the appropriate pocket.   Pocket patterns appear on the next page.

FILL THE POCKETS

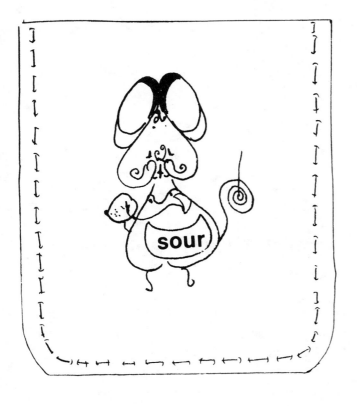

sour

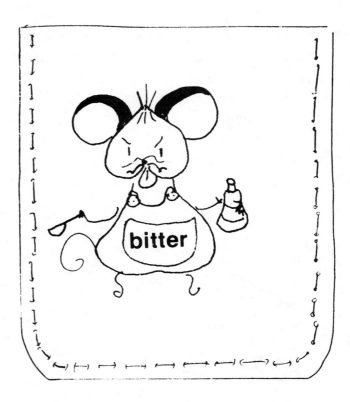

bitter

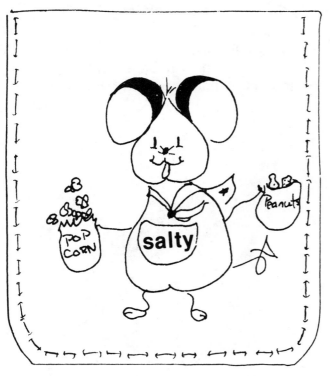

salty

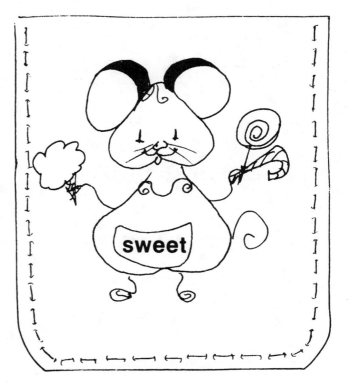

sweet

CARROT SALAD

Scrub the carrots well and leave the skins on. Grate them into a big bowl. Add a scoop full of raisins. Pour some lemon juice over the mixture. Add some honey or corn syrup until the salad tastes just right.

Enjoy!

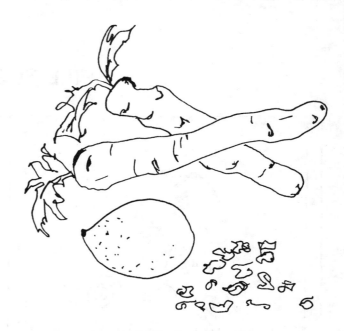

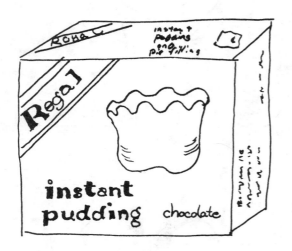

PAINT WITH PUDDING

Have the children bring their favorite flavor of instant pudding to school. Follow the directions on the pudding mix box.

Before painting, have a tasting time when the children can taste the different flavors.

When ready to paint give each child a 12" X 18" piece of finger-paint paper and one or two tablespoons of instant pudding. Have fun.

TASTING MOUTH

Tasting steak is really great,

but if I had my way,

I'd eat chocolate cake,

All night and all day.

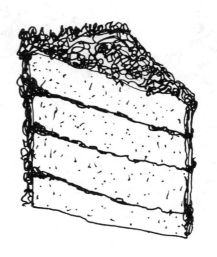

Draw a picture of your very favorite food.

GROUPING - SORTING

You will need a cookie sheet or large tray for this activity. Cut three sheets of paper, one yellow, one red and one green, and place on the tray covering the surface entirely.

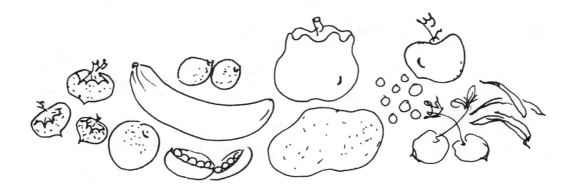

Also on the tray place a variety of fruits and vegetables. The student's task is to place each item on the corresponding color of paper.

WHAT'S ON THE TRAY?

Have several fresh fruits and vegetables on a tray. The children should identify the fruits and vegetables. Younger children can identify the fruits and vegetables by naming each orally. Older children can match a word card with each item. After a discussion, have a sampling party. Then discuss the taste of each fruit or vegetable. Have extra pieces of the fruits and vegetables available so that every child gets to taste each.

Suggested items for tray:

apple	peanut	cherry	orange
tomato	plum	pear	pickle
berries	peach	olive	green pepper
grapes	carrot	pineapple	peas
cauliflower	lettuce	cabbage	beans
corn	melon	celery	raisins
parsley			

A CHANT - WHO STOLE THE COOKIE?

The teacher and the students take turns chanting the words to this poem. Encourage expressive chanting. Use the names of the students participating instead of the names included in the sample below.

Susie asks: "Who stole the cookie from the cookie jar?"

Bill answers: "Ann stole the cookie from the cookie jar."

Ann says: "Who, me?"

Bill answers: "Yes, you."

Ann says: "Not me!"

Bill asks: "Then who?"

Ann says: "John stole the cookie from the cookie jar."

John answers: "Who, me?" etc.

Repeat until everyone has had a turn.

RIDDLES - GUESS WHAT?

In a riddle form describe a food. Be sure to include color, size and taste.

Examples:

It is yellow.
It is smaller
    than an orange.
It is sour.
What is it?

(lemon)

It is red.
It grows on a vine.
It has many many
    little seeds.
What is it?

(tomato)

It is long.
It is yellow and brown
    on the outside and white
    on the inside.
Monkeys like these.
What is it ?

(banana)

FIND THE BONE

Use three different colors of crayons. Trace a
path so each dog can get to the bone.

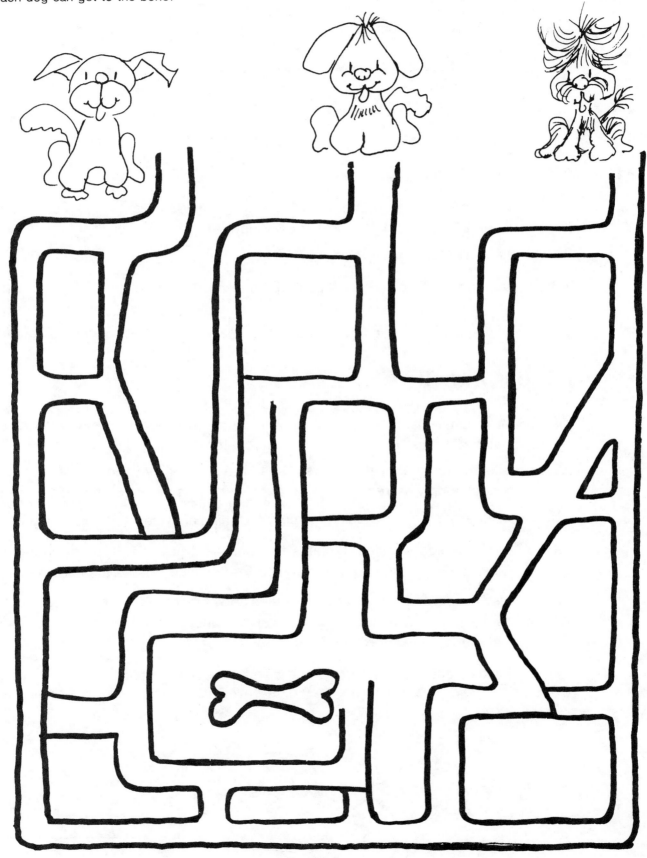

HOW DO WE SMELL THINGS?

TOPIC CONCEPTS TO BE DEVELOPED:

1. The nose is the part of the body that is used for smelling.

2. The odors of things help us to identify them.

3. Smelling is one of our senses.

LARGE GROUP ACTIVITIES:

1. Walk through your school building and identify smells. A walk can also be taken in the neighborhood surrounding the school.

2. Take a field trip to a bakery.

3. During storytime read poems and stories about smells. Films and filmstrips could also be shown.

4. During a craft period have the students make gift sachets or drawer sachets.

SMALL GROUP ACTIVITIES:

1. Make smelly jars. Baby food jars are a good size for this activity. Students match word cards with the smell encountered in each jar.

2. Use scratch and sniff stickers. These are inexpensive and available at most school supply stores. This is an excellent way to reward students.

3. Create and play vocabulary games, matching activities and sorting activities.

4. Burn scented candles. Discuss the smell and how it is kept in the candle. Room deodorizers can also be used for this kind of smelling activity.

5. Display and sniff a variety of perfumes and colognes. Can the various scents be detected? What are the various smells encountered? How do fragrances that men and women use differ?

6. Make a collage of people's and animal's noses. Display and discuss. How are they similar? How are they different? Do all creatures' noses do an equal job?

DRAWER SACHET

Materials needed:

      bars of scented soap   tempera paint
      white glue   various colors of yarn
      straight pins   various colors of felt

Directions:

Smooth off the trade name on a bar of soap with a damp sponge. Paint on a face with tempera paint mixed with an equal part of white glue.

Cut hair from yarn or a hat from felt and glue or pin to the bar of soap. Short length straight pins work well. Be sure they are not too long.

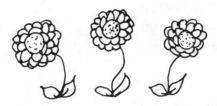

POPCORN FLOWERS

Materials needed:

      popped corn   white glue
      powdered tempera   pencil
      crayons   12" X 18" paper

Directions:
While popping the corn be sure to discuss the odor, the sounds, and of course, do some tasting.

On the large sheet of construction paper have the child sketch some large flowers. Color all the picture with crayons except the petals of the flowers. The petals should be outlined.

Using glue, fill each petal shape with popped corn that has been colored with powdered tempera. (Place a tablespoon of colored tempra and 2-3 cups of popped corn in a grocery bag. Shake to color.)

GIFT SACHETS

Materials needed:

    perfume
    blotting paper
    crayons
    tag board
    paste or glue

Directions:

Place a drop of perfume on a one inch square of blotting paper. Then glue the blotting paper onto a larger piece of paper decorated with the child's crayon drawing. The completed sachet can then be placed in an envelope and addressed to the person to whom it is intended.

These gifts are nice to place in closets and cupboards.

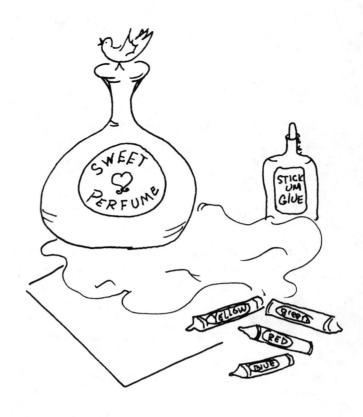

SMELL TRAY

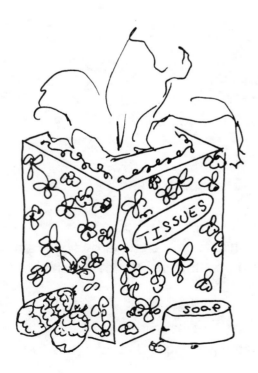

The object of this activity is to be able to identify by smell as many items as possible that have been placed on the tray. Smells can be compared and discussed. You may wish to graph the results. Which smells were easiest to identify? Why?

Items that could be used include:

magazine	newspaper
tissue	cork
soap	leather
fur	cedarwood
incense	pine cone
foam rubber	carpet
linoleum	evergreen

PICTURE CARDS FOR GOOD SMELLS - BAD SMELLS

Cut out, along the dotted lines, the picture cards and the word cards found on the next page. Place all the bad smell picture cards in the bad smells section on this page. Put all the good smells cards in the good smells section on this page.

GOOD SMELLS	BAD SMELLS

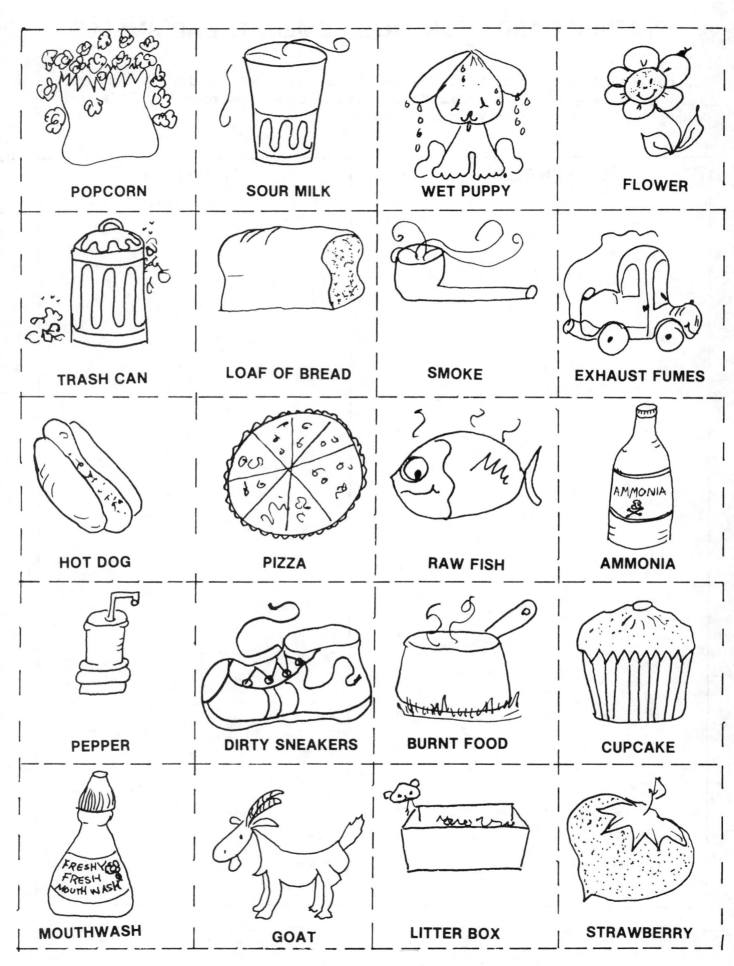

POPCORN	SOUR MILK	WET PUPPY	FLOWER
TRASH CAN	LOAF OF BREAD	SMOKE	EXHAUST FUMES
HOT DOG	PIZZA	RAW FISH	AMMONIA
PEPPER	DIRTY SNEAKERS	BURNT FOOD	CUPCAKE
MOUTHWASH	GOAT	LITTER BOX	STRAWBERRY

GOOD SMELLS

First, color the picture. Then cut it apart on the dotted lines. Reassemble the picture.

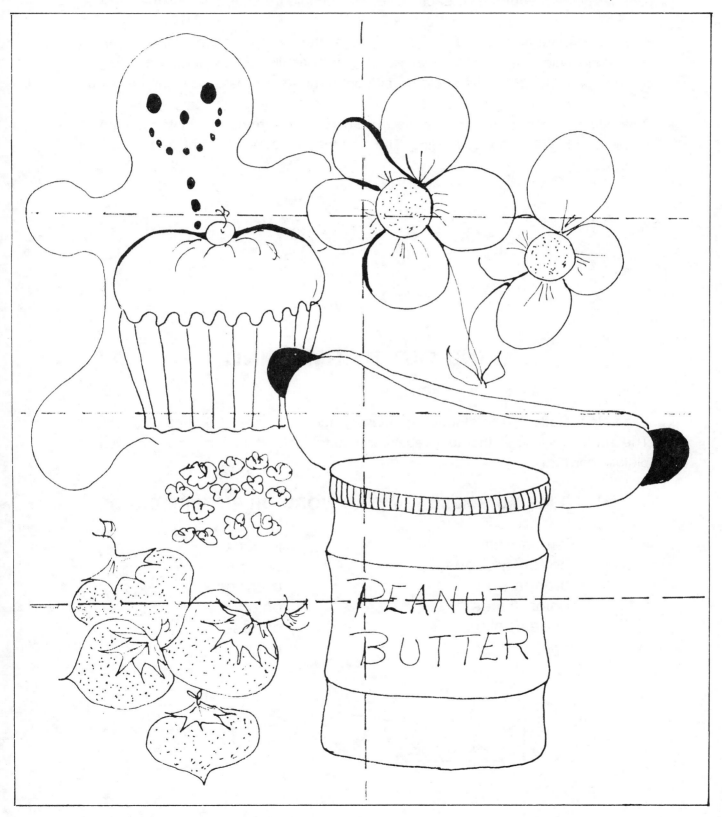

"SMELLY" JARS

You will need several small jars. Baby food jars or pill containers will work well. In each jar place a cotton ball. Each cotton ball should be dampened with an aroma.

Perfume, peppermint, coffee, cocoa, peanut butter, shaving lotion, ammonia, onion juice, lemon juice, paint thinner, vanilla, beer and gasoline are among the smells that can be used. Some spices could be hidden in the cotton balls and also be used.

On the lid of each jar glue or tape the word card or picture card to match the aroma inside the jar. Then, mix up the lids. The task for the student is to place the correct lid on each jar.

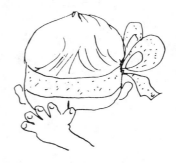

FIND OUT BY SMELLING

Blindfold a student. The student will identify items by smell. Take the blindfold off. The student will smell the items again and match each item with a correct word or picture card.

ITEMS TO SMELL	WORD OR PICTURE CARDS
lemon rind	lemon
coffee grounds	coffee
orange rind	orange
onion flakes	onion
cheese slice	cheese
rose	flower

THINGS
I LIKE
TO SMELL

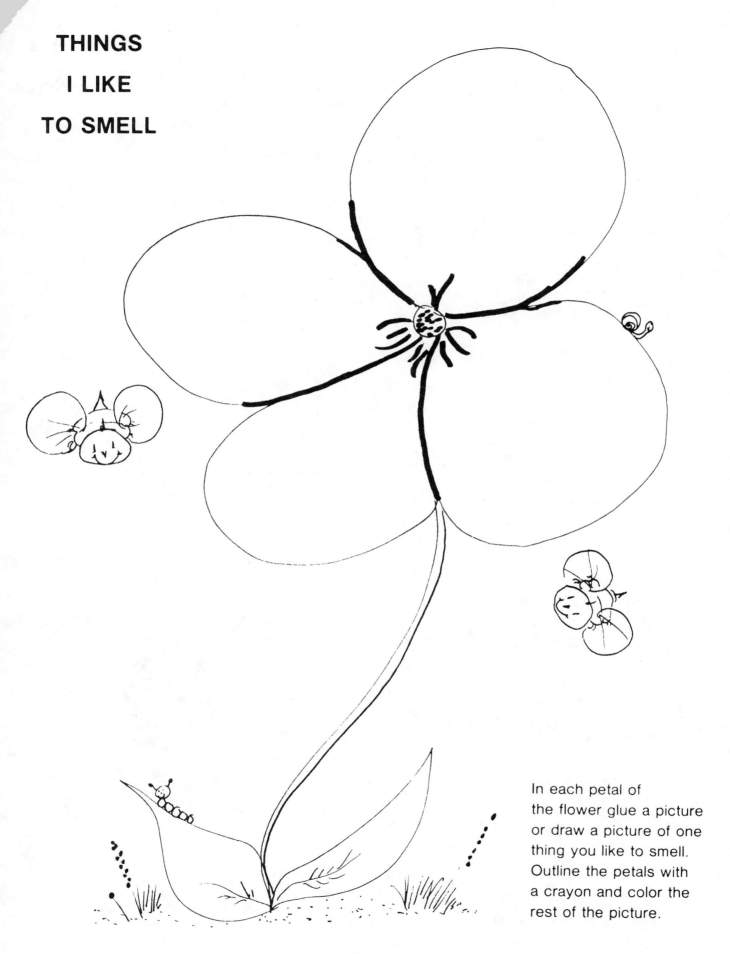

In each petal of
the flower glue a picture
or draw a picture of one
thing you like to smell.
Outline the petals with
a crayon and color the
rest of the picture.

PINOCCHIO

Draw Pinocchio's nose.
On the nose paste pictures
    or draw pictures of things
    that can be smelled.
Color the picture.
Read the riddle.
Answer the riddle.

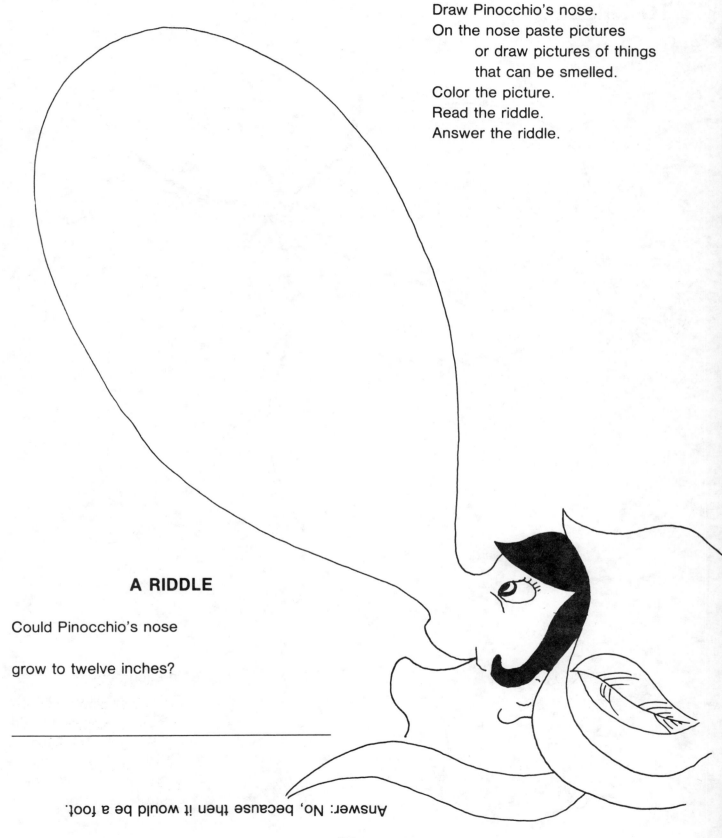

A RIDDLE

Could Pinocchio's nose

grow to twelve inches?

_____

Answer: No, because then it would be a foot.

THE NOSE KNOWS

The elephant's nose is long and gray,

He uses it to smell the fresh _____.

Draw a picture of something else for the elephant to smell.

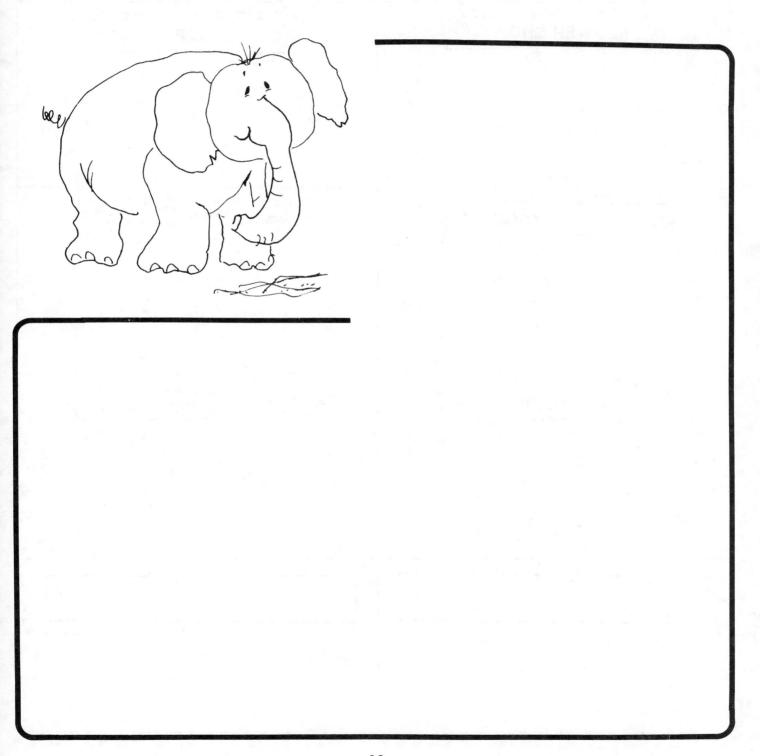

A SWELL SMELL TRIP

Take a smell trip. Visit a lot of places. What would you smell if you went to the places listed below? Draw your answers. There are two blank places so you can add a couple more.

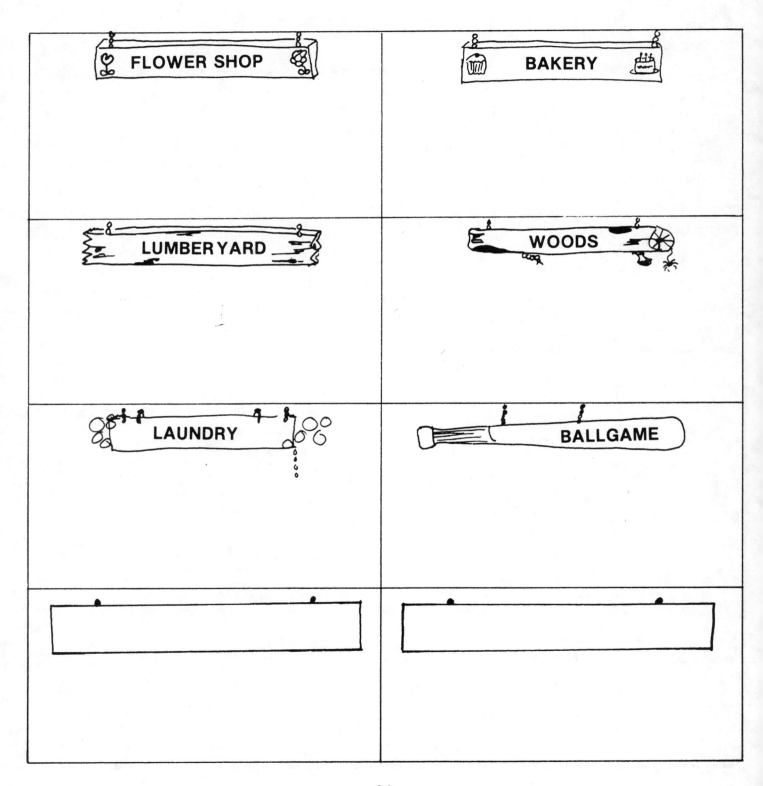